CONTROL YOUR BLOOD

SUGAR WITH HEALTHY FOODS

BY

DR.TYLER SMITH

TABLE OF CONTENT

CHAPTER ONE

INTRODUCTION

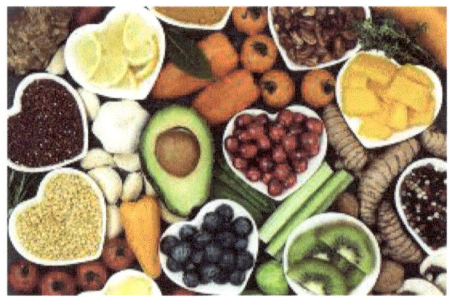

One strategy to help lower or manage

blood sugar levels is to choose foods

with a low glycemic index (GI). The GI

calculates the impact of various foods on blood sugar levels.

The greatest foods and drinks for diabetics are those that the body absorbs gradually because they prevent blood sugar spikes and troughs.

People who want to control their blood sugar levels should choose foods with low or medium GI scores. A variety of bread types have high GI ratings and may cause blood sugar levels to increase. Therefore, many are better off avoided by those who have diabetes. To make sure a meal is balanced, people can also match meals with low and high GI values.

Certain advantages come from controlling blood sugar levels, including increased vitality and happiness as well as a lower risk of developing certain chronic diseases. A healthy lifestyle that includes regular exercise, drinking plenty of water, and eating balanced meals will naturally maintain blood sugar levels while also providing extra health benefits including lowered cholesterol and enhanced gut health.

CHAPTER TWO

CONSUME CARBOHYDRATES LAST

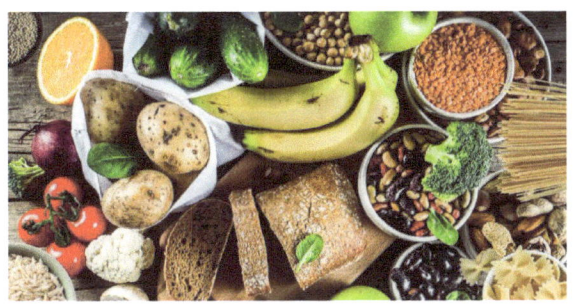

Even though it might not be feasible to follow this strategy at every meal, research indicates that eating calories after veggies lowers the amount of sugar in the blood after meals.

In a single research study, 16 people with diabetes type 2 consumed the same food on distinct occasions in one of three different orders: calories first, accompanied by vegetable and protein sources just ten minutes later; proteins and vegetables before anything else, followed by calories 10 minutes thereafter; or all nutrients simultaneously.

Just prior to meals and every 30 minutes following them for for a maximum of three hours, blood sugar, insulin, and other measurements were obtained. The consumption of calories at the end of a meal as opposed to the beginning considerably reduced glucose levels in the blood, according to research

Similar to a further analysis of the scientific research, the order in which you consume your meals affects how much sugar stays in your system after a meal. Experts recommend eating abundant-water and nutrients from fibre first (such veggies), followed by foods with significant protein content, oils/fats, last carefully assimilated whole, complex carbohydrate sources, and then basic carbohydrates or foods high in sugar molecules.Blood glucose is created during digestion from carbohydrates and carbs. Starches are also referred to as complex carbohydrates, whilst sugars are referred to as simple carbs. Consider choosing healthy carbohydrates like: Fruits,Vegetables,complete grains.

legumes, including peas and beans.

dairy items like milk and cheese that are low in fat.

Avoid less nutritious sources of carbs, such as items with added fats, sweets, or sodium.

CHAPTER THREE

MAKE YOUR MEALS RICHER IN SOLUBLE FIBRE.

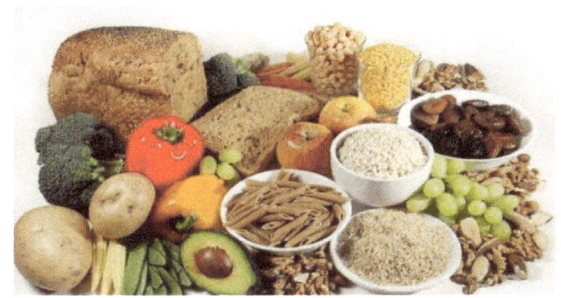

A specific kind of carbohydrates known as fibre is not digested and released into blood vessels through the gut. Consequently, the fibre in meals high in carbohydrates won't trigger a spike in blood glucose levels. Particularly water-soluble fibre limits the breakdown of food, which causes the ingested calories to enter into the blood stream even more slowly. The blood sugar surge that follows a meal is lessened as a result. Research revealed that including soluble fibre in a sweet beverage significantly reduced total blood sugar levels. Higher soluble fibre content in morning meals, whether from foods that are high in fibre or a soluble fibre nutrient supplements, resulted in a decrease in the blood's glucose levels after the meal .

All the components of plant foods that your body cannot digest or absorb are considered dietary fibre. The gradual digestion of meals by fibre aids in blood sugar regulation. Some of the foods high in fibre include:

Vegetables, Fruits, Nuts, legumes, including peas and beans.

complete grains, seeds, lentils, peas, apples, bananas, oats, avocados,

Brussels sprouts, are also packed with compounds that contain soluble fiber.

CHAPTER FOUR

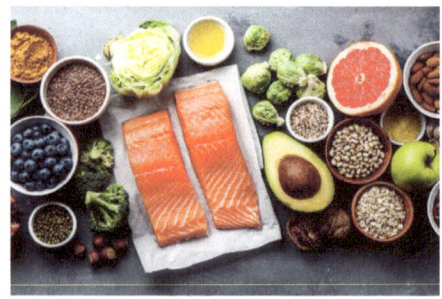

EAT BREAKFAST RICH IN PROTEIN.

A protein-rich breakfast may contribute to all-day reductions in blood sugar levels following meals. According to short research of 12 healthy adults, those who ate a breakfast with a lot of protein had lower post-meal blood sugar levels than those who typically have a low-protein breakfast. This was true for all three meals of the day.

CHAPTER FIVE

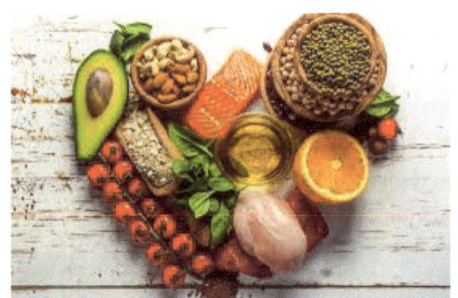

GIVE INTERMITTENT FASTING A TRY.

For slimming down and other well-being advantages, such as controlling blood sugar, intermittent fasting (IF) has gained popularity. There are many methods to implement (IF,) but according to some studies, it may be preferable to consume the majority of your calorie intake in morning and noon and have a lighter meal earlier in the evening to control your glucose levels specifically. Even in healthy individuals, eating later in the evening makes it harder for blood sugar to levels to regulate after meals. Despite the particular form of IF intervention, study reviews indicated that (IF) benefited the physical health for persons with high blood sugar concentrations and high cholesterol levels.

Developments in haemoglobin A1C, also known as HbA1c, a test taken from the blood that determines how much sugar is present in the blood over the three months prior to the test, were among them.

CHAPTER SIX

PICK WHOLE GRAINS INSTEAD OF REFINED GRAINS.

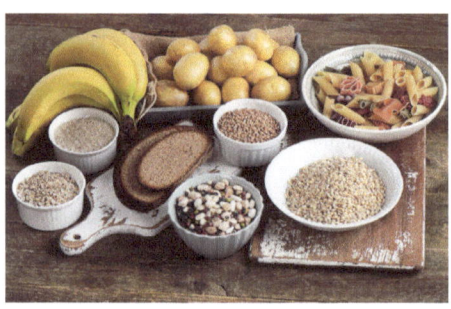

In particular, when it comes to how they impact your blood sugar levels, not all carbohydrates are created equal. When compared to refined carbohydrate items after a meal, the consumption of whole grains continuously improved blood glucose levels, . Pick whole grains instead of grains that are refined. Among the many varieties of whole grains are:

brown rice and amaranth, Barley

Buckwheat Millet Oats Popcorn

Wild rice Sorghum Quinoa

Examples of refined grains include:

 white rice, most white breads , corn grits. White flour and food with refined grains includes cakes ,pastries and crackers.

CHAPTER SEVEN

AFTER MEALS GO FOR A WALK

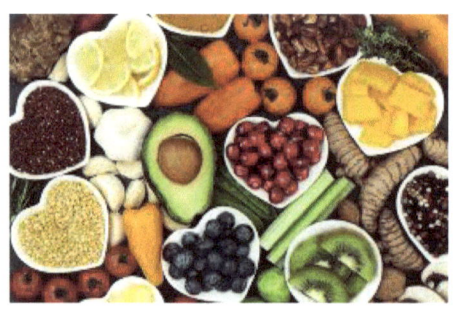

Walking after eating enables your body to use current carbohydrate intake to fuel muscle action, which lowers your blood sugar levels after meals. Additionally, walking helps insulin operate more efficiently to remove sugar from your blood.

In a research study conducted in 21 healthy young volunteers were divided into two different categories to examine the effects of walking. After meals with varying levels of carbs, the first group went on brisk 30-minute walks. After consuming a mixed lunch or a beverage high in carbohydrates, another group went on brisk 30-minute walks. Researchers discovered that vigorous exercise significantly lowered both groups' post-meal blood sugar peaks.

Even standing rather than sitting after meals resulted in decreased post-meal blood sugar levels, according to a 2022 study, although mild intensity walking was more efficient.

CHAPTER EIGHT

WORK ON YOUR STRENGTH

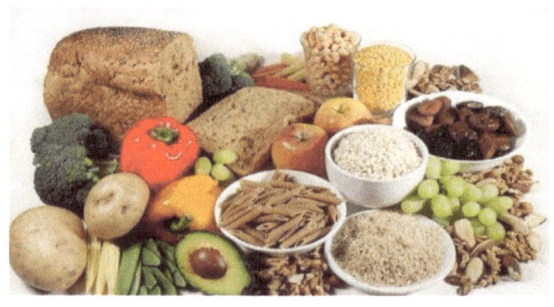

Performing resistance exercises can help regulate blood sugar levels in addition to enhancing muscle and strength. One session of resistance training before a meal significantly decreased post-meal their blood sugar levels in 10 inactive males with obesity and prediabetes, according to a 2021 study.

In a second, smaller trial, eight persons with type 2 diabetes were examined to determine the effects of different activities on blood sugar levels following a meal. They were 15 minutes of circuit resistance training, 30 minutes of uninterrupted sitting, 30 minutes of walking and cardiovascular activity. Despite the fact that resistance training required the least time investment, research has shown that all forms of exercise improved blood sugar management after meals

- RECOMMENDATIONS FOR BEGINNERS WEIGHTLIFTING
- Consider the your bodyweight first.
- Establish your form.
- Make an equipment purchase.
- Before you begin, prepare your muscles.
- Choose the proper weight to lift.

- When you first begin, keep performing the same motions every day.
- If you can, squeeze in a post-workout stretch.

CHAPTER NINE

EXPAND YOUR CONSUMPTION OF

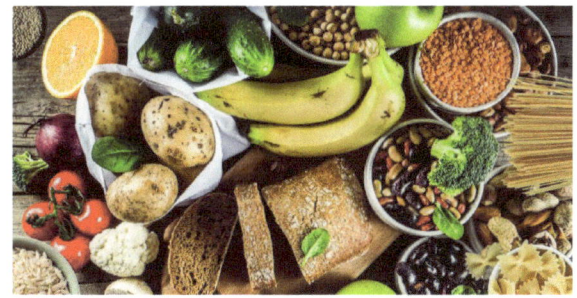

PULSES

Beans, lentils, peas, and chickpeas come under the category of pulses. This food category contains an exceptional blend of protein and carbohydrates with high fibre content, as well as a number of essential minerals and vitamins.

Consume a greater amount of pulse to enhance both post-meal blood sugar control and long-term management, including HbA1c readings, according to a research review published in 2022 for persons who have or don't have diabetes of any kind.

Add pulses to salads, soups, vegetable chilli, tacos, and curries. Choose pulse-based dips like hummus and bean dip as well as pulse-based pastas like chickpea or lentil penne.

CHAPTER TEN

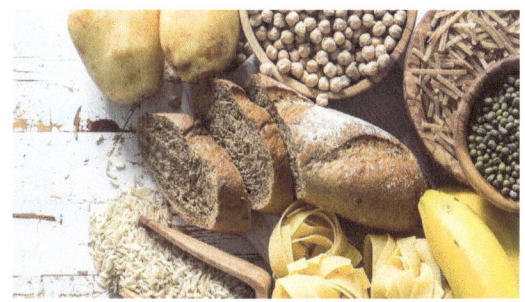

BREAKFAST SHOULD BE PROTEIN-RICH

A protein-rich breakfast may lower blood sugar levels after meals all through each day. One short research of 12 individuals in good health discovered that those who ate a high protein breakfasts experienced lesser post-meal levels of blood sugar than those who typically have a lower protein breakfast. Compared to the average breakfast's 18% of calories from protein, the high protein breakfast's 60% of calories were made up of this macronutrient. Don't overlook veggies when seeking out extra protein. Those who consumed more foods that are made from plants had a smaller chance of prediabetes, type 2 diabetes, and insulin resistance, a condition which occurs when insulin doesn't operate as it should to remove sugar from the blood, according to a significant population-based study involving more than seven thousand individuals over almost eight years.

You might improve your health and the environment by consuming more plant-based protein and less animal protein. Plant-based proteins have several advantages which includes;More dietary fibre And nutrients,minimal Or Nonexistent Saturated Fat, which Is

Linked to heart disease,no or little sodium, lower likelihood of Attack and cardiac disease ,lowered Risk Of Obesity, Hypertension, Type 2 Diabetes, And Certain Malignancies,reduces greenhouse gases and other emissions of pollutants.

CHAPTER ELEVEN

CONSUME MORE AVOCADO

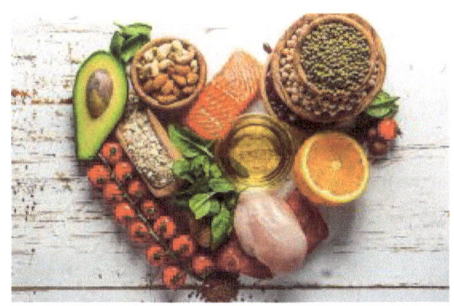

Healthy fats, vitamins, minerals, antioxidants, and fibre are all abundant in avocados. It has been proven that incorporating them into meals will help control blood sugar levels.

In a research study conducted in three calorie-equal meals with either no avocado, half an avocado, or a whole avocado were compared in 31 overweight or obese participants. When compared to meals without avocado, those that included a half or a whole avocado had lower post-meal blood glucose levels and better blood flow.

It was discovered that throughout a six-year period, people who regularly ate avocado had a lower risk of developing type 2 diabetes than people who didn't, particularly if they had prediabetes at the start of the trial.

CHAPTER TWELVE

WEAR A CONTINUOUS GLUCOSE MONITOR (CGM)

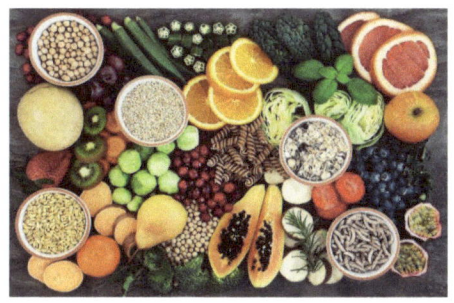

A Continuous Glucose Monitor should be worn by Individuals who suffer from diabetes have typically utilised continuous blood sugar devices, or CGMs. But users who just want to keep track and regulate more effectively their blood sugar levels have become more and more accustomed to using the devices.

The intercellular sugar level, which is the sugar found in the fluid within the cells, is measured by CGMs using apps that are synced to sensors (usually located on the back of the arm).

CHAPTER THIRTEEN

CONSUME AND DRINK MORE

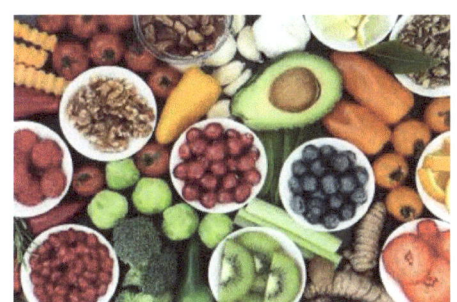

FERMENTED FOODS

The process of fermenting is anaerobic breakdown of carbohydrates by yeast or microbial agents to produce alcohol or acids that are organic. Kefir, kombucha, sauerkraut, tempeh, natto, miso, kimchi, and sourdough bread are examples of fermented foods. Science indicates that fermented meals may decrease the absorption of carbohydrates, which results in lower post-meal blood sugar levels in addition to promoting digestive health. Science indicates that fermented meals may decrease the absorption of carbohydrates, which results in lower post-meal blood sugar levels in addition to promoting digestive health.

Additionally demonstrated to lessen inflammation, a risk factor for type 2 diabetes, are fermented foods.

CHAPTER FOURTEEN

LIMIT YOUR CONSUMPTION OF ADDED

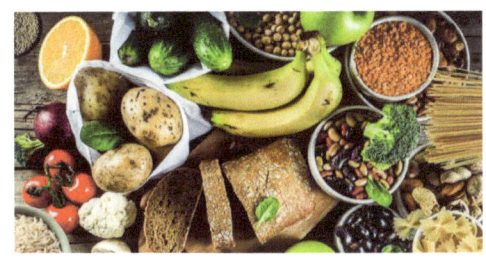

SUGAR

A food item has added sugar if it has been sweetened by the manufacturer or if you personally add it, such as by stirring sugar into your morning cup of coffee.Blood sugar levels rise as a result of added sugar's rapid absorption into the bloodstream. Additionally, consuming too much added sugar over time raises the chance of developing diabetes as well as heart disease, dementia, Alzheimer's, obesity, high blood pressure, and several types of cancer According to other study, the overall incidence of type 2 diabetes and prediabetes is reduced by about 50% when added sugar intake is limited to less than 5% of total calories. Women should consume not more than 25 grammes (or six teaspoons) of added sugar daily, while males should consume not more than 36 grammes (or nine teaspoons).

According to other study, the prevalence of type 2 diabetes and prediabetes is reduced by about 50% when added sugar intake is limited to less than 5% of total calories.

CHAPTER FIFTEEN

CUT BACK ON SUGAR SUBSTITUTES

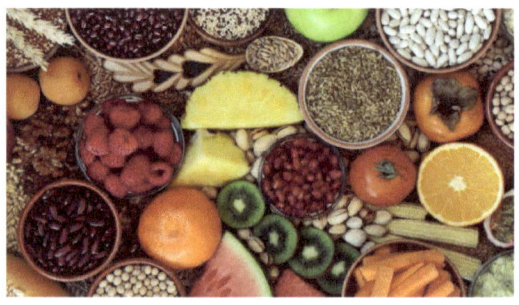

Sugar replacements are not an effective choice for long-term control of blood sugar or lowering the risk of developing diabetes, despite the fact that they don't rapidly boost blood sugar levels like additional sugars do. This is because it has been demonstrated that artificial sugars increase insulin levels, which can eventually result in insulin resistance and reduce insulin's ability to effectively remove sugar from the blood

The World Health Organisation (WHO) dissuaded the use of non-sugar sweeteners in 2023 in order to control body weight or lower the risk of disease. In accordance with a scientific assessment, the organisation said that long-term usage of non-sugar sweeteners may have unfavourable impacts, such as an elevated risk of type 2 diabetes and cardiovascular disease.

CHAPTER SIXTEEN

BOOST YOUR VITAMIN D INTAKE

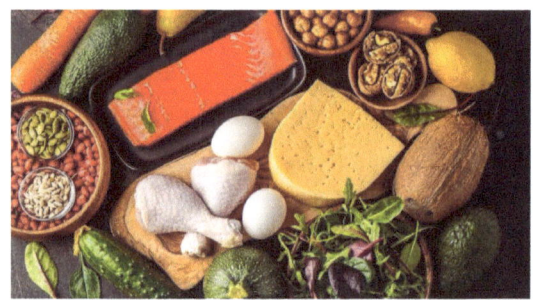

Using the American Diabetes Association, approximately four in ten persons are vitamin D deficient, which can have a detrimental effect on blood sugar management .It's also critical to note that excessive vitamin D intake can result in excessively high blood calcium levels, which over time can harm bones, soft tissues, and the kidneys In individuals with type 2 diabetes and insufficient vitamin D. In persons with prediabetes and low vitamin D levels, other studies have indicated that a vitamin D supplement decreased the chance of developing diabetes by 15% and raised the likelihood of normalising blood sugar management by 30%. Before taking a supplement, if you're unclear of your vitamin D status, talk to your doctor about having your blood level checked.

CHAPTER SEVENTEEN

KEEP YOURSELF HYDRATED

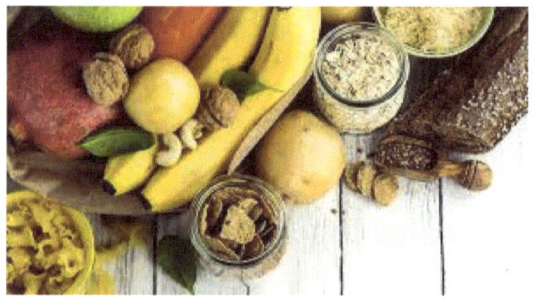

In comparison to those who don't drink enough water, a Prospective study found that those who do appear to be healthier, experience fewer chronic diseases, and live longer. A benefit of maintaining proper hydration may be the control of blood sugar. A review of the literature published in 2021 revealed an association between drinking more water and a lower risk of diabetes who have type 2 diabetes fluids.